PRAISE FOR THE POETRY OF RAFAEL CAMPO

The Enemy (2007)

"Rafael Campo writes tough, questioning, rueful, exquisite, true-hearted poems that resist nostalgia while testing the transformative power of beauty. In perfectly wrought poem after poem, he explores the 'honor' of sacrifice and the breadth of human fidelities. The Enemy is surely Campo's best book yet."—ELIZABETH ALEXANDER, Yale University

"Rafael Campo is one of the most significant poets writing in America today. In exploring the complexities of his position—Cuban American, gay, Harvard grad, physician, scrupulous observer of himself, of others, and of the worlds we inhabit—he has produced a richly textured, layered body of work, distinguished for its mastery of, and wrestling with, poetic form, as well as for its courage, compassion, and clarity. Hybrid—a mix of memory and desire, trust and fear, anger and love—his work has always been death-haunted yet he speaks for what is alive and healing in American culture."—ALICIA SUSKIN OSTRIKER, author of No Heaven

"Rafael Campo's The Enemy moves with naturalness, speed, and balance between experiences of domestic love—a couple of gay men, celebrating rites of daily ordinariness—and scenes from a doctor's life. We turn to Campo for frankness, freshness, and the tang of truth, and we are rewarded."—ROSANNA WARREN, author of Departure

"[Campo] writes of music and celebrates the erotic. He has awe for the mysterious and a familiarity with despair, and he catches frequent hints of God's presence. In this book, there are tiresome days in the clinic and patients who are near death but who will not die. . . . [His] poems show how medicine can best be of service in the absence of cures or quick fixes, and how medical professionals can best be present, mindfully and emotionally, during moments of human suffering."
—HEATHER A. BURNS, The New England Journal of Medicine

T0204311

Landscape with Human Figure (2002)

"Rafael Campo is an accomplished formalist. I hugely enjoy watching him skitter from sestina to pantoum, sonnet to rhymed couplets, to say nothing of his own nonce forms devised as the situation suggests."
—MAXINE KUMIN

"*Landscape with Human Figure* is a striking achievement. I am moved, as his readers are sure to be, by Campo's wisdom, maturity, depth, heart, and range of experience."—GRACE SCHULMAN

"Campo writes restless, worldly narrative poems, often rhyming, that take—and unapologetically engage—the world as it presents itself. . . . [His] insouciant, call-them-as-I-seem-them descriptions . . . are luminous, addressing the ravages of AIDS, particularly, with care and respect."—*Publishers Weekly*

"Ambitious, elegant poems. . . . Campo's clear gaze, generous heart, and great skill combine to create a resonant and often romantic collection of poems, one that locates and celebrates all our shared 'outsider' hearts."—KEVIN RIORDAN, *Philadelphia Gay News*

"Physician Rafael Campo confirms his status as one of America's most important poets."—*Hispanic Outlook*

"Campo writes compelling poems . . . probing relationships between doctor and patient, between a patient's case 'history' and the cultural mainstream, between an immigrant family and aspirations to study medicine, between sexuality and the restraint of lovers. Not unlike Chekhov, another physician-author, the steady-eyed Campo comes to terms with the darkest of human problems . . . by fusing empathy and clinical accuracy. Strengthened by his hands-on knowledge of healing and suffering and kept gentle by bearing his burdens with grace, Campo asserts that, despite 'the harrowed world . . . we are together, we are here to stay.'"—FRANK ALLEN, *Library Journal*

Diva (1999)

"Extraordinary meditations on illness and the healing power of words."—*Lambda Literary Foundation*

"Campo writes mordant lyrics of dark love that displace trite expectations of what sonnets or *canciones* should accomplish. . . . [His] work hastens our absorption of what initially seems alien."—JERRY W. WARD JR., *The Washington Post Book World*

"A virtuoso display. . . . Campo is a master of image. . . . His poems are revealing and courageous."—JAY A. LIVESON, MD, JAMA: *The Journal of the American Medical Association*

"Rafael Campo is perhaps our most distinguished physician-poet since William Carlos Williams."—DAVID BERGMAN, *The Gay and Lesbian Review Worldwide*

"I know of no poet writing today with more courage and compassion than Rafael Campo. Like the practicing physician that he is, Campo writes poems that heal artfully—or honestly face the impossibility of healing. Here we find sonnets for the damned, songs for the dying, the insistence on empathy for a prostitute with AIDS on a Boston street corner. There is the unforgiving squint of a mother rejecting her gay son. Yet there is a soaring lyricism in these poems, epiphany and redemption, a celebration of bloodstained, stubborn life as it bursts forth. The poems of Rafael Campo inspire that sharp breath of recognition. He has all my gratitude and admiration."—MARTÍN ESPADA, author of *Imagine the Angels of Bread*

What the Body Told (1996)

"Rafael Campo is one of the most gifted and accomplished younger poets writing in English. More than that, he is a writer engaged in several of the pivotal struggles/issues of our era, and what he has to say about them is 'news that stays news.'"—MARILYN HACKER

ALTERNATIVE MEDICINE

ALTERNATIVE

MEDICINE

RAFAEL CAMPO

DUKE UNIVERSITY PRESS

Durham and London · 2014

Library of Congress Cataloging-in-

Publication Data

Campo, Rafael.

Alternative medicine / Rafael Campo.

pages cm

ISBN 978-0-8223-5573-1 (cloth : alk. paper)

ISBN 978-0-8223-5587-8 (pbk. : alk. paper)

I. Title.

PS3553.A4883A48 2013

811'.54—dc23

2013030385

CONTENTS

III. PLONK

ACKNOWLEDGMENTS

I am very grateful to the editors of the following journals and
periodicals, who published some of the poems in this collection,
sometimes in slightly different forms:

Bellevue Literary Review
The Common
Columbia Poetry Review
Gay and Lesbian Review Worldwide
Harvard Divinity Bulletin
Harvard Review
Journal of the Medical Humanities
Iron Horse Literary Review
Massachusetts Review
Measure
North American Review
Plume
Poetry Northwest
Poets.org
The Progressive
Slate.com
Seneca Review
Southwest Review
Sugar House Review
The Threepenny Review
upstreet
The Yale Review

"Recent Past Events" was cited as a Commended Poem in the
2012 Hippocrates International Open Prize competition and was
first published in the Hippocrates Prize Anthology 2012.

I.

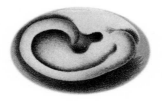

HAVANA

Havana

When we were six or seven, Dad would quiz us
on the capitals of the world, me and my kid brothers
who didn't even know our own address. We lived
in New Jersey, not Cuba, and our ignorance
seemed like the reason we would never,
ever go there. So I tried to memorize the names
of the stars printed on my National Geographic
Map of the World: L-I-M-A was the capital of Peru,
not just a kind of bean I hated; I wondered if Peru
was anything like Cuba. I wondered if I would ever see
what I imagined were the horrible, muddy streets
of Helsinki, which sounded like a place where sinners
like me would be punished, sucked into the earth
for good; even Ottawa, in our nice neighbor Canada,
seemed incomprehensibly far away. It was always
at dinnertime when he'd start in on us: *Who knows
the capital of Burma?* I stared into my succotash,
pushing it around and around with my fork,
sure that children there were starving, dying
of starvation in a city whose name I didn't even know.
One night, with the distant stars flickering outside
the steamed-up kitchen windows, he asked,
Does anyone here know the capital of Cuba?
Every bone in my body ached with the answer,
the one place in the world I most wanted to visit,
the one place in the world whose name
was always impossible for me to remember.

My Kind of Love Poem

Unluckily, the day begins: a bomb
has detonated in Mumbai. Again,
we ask ourselves: Is this what we've become?
Unluckily, the night has eyes. A train
makes music of the city's sleeplessness
again; a baby shrieks with hunger or
the need to have its diaper changed. Unless
he finds a job, the man who lives next door
will have to go on unemployment. Bombs
explode in other places, ruining
other lives, scarring other faces. Crumbs
form constellations in my sink. The ring
of doorbells, telephones, and certain phrases:
The night dies. Unlucky Saturn rises.

A History of Poetry

The first poem was the sound of a tree
falling in the vast wilderness.

Soon, human beings roamed all the earth.
They scrawled poems on the walls of caves.

Thousands of years more passed. When God
made himself known, poems became prayers.

Then poetry evolved into an art,
its music mimicking the beating heart.

Tired of airs, poets wrote new poems that
broke the rules
                        for a while, anyway.

Even those poems grew old. Ergo, poetry
came to mean that meaning came. (What the #@!!?)

Now, it's only a matter of time before poetry
on the Internet becomes self-aware.

The poetry of the future will destroy its masters.
In the aftermath, as in the beginning, none

will be sure it even still exists. Only then
will it remember what it always was: everything

the survivors might one day understand.

Wilhelmina Shakespeare

Blond hair, blue eyes, buck teeth: we taunted you
because of your intelligence. You loved
to read, and secretly I envied how
you gave yourself to poetry, alone
beneath the shade a mango tree provided.
We dubbed you "Wilhelmina Shakespeare" when
we locked you in the basement, proving force
could triumph over wisdom. "She's a witch!"
we bellowed as we torched your diary—
but nothing we could do would make you cry.
You knew the scientific names of rocks;
you tried to teach me Spanish once, but I
responded to your questions in pig Latin.
At night, when all my other cousins watched
reruns of Hawaii 5-o, I'd sneak
away to spy on you. Out on the porch,
you'd be there with your sketch pad studying
the moths that crowded the bare lightbulb, starved
for that dim light, that least illumination.
Your features softened as I gazed at you:
I understood my insignificance
as I saw it was possible to know
the beauty in even the plainest things.

The Common Mental Health Disorders of Immigrants

I. POST-TRAUMATIC STRESS DISORDER

My nephew watches the survivalist
on television drink his own dark piss,
eat spiders, clamber down a waterfall—
he's white and blue-eyed, good-looking, agile.
He makes a shelter from his parachute.
Behind him, no one chases after him,
besides the desert's looming black eagle
as silent as a shadow, bored as God.
He doesn't hope to have a better life.
His thirst is momentary, hunger an
imagined state; his sister doesn't sell
herself to British tourists so her kids
can have school books. Dogs barking distantly,
flashlight beams needling the night, nowhere
to go but in the steps of those before.
That night, they ate cold beans from cans; they drank
the water pooled inside a cast-off tire.
They left the little girl with diarrhea
asleep beneath a rocky ledge. No one
found a parachute to make a tent, or
drank his own piss in order to survive.

II. DEPRESSION

She smokes, as if she could inhale it all
and make it vanish: all the poisonous
miasmas, all the mysterious dreams,
the tears my grandfather shed, where she hid
while soldiers smashed the grand piano, black
as a deep lake, to pieces. Now, her house
is small and spare: telenovelas blare,
though the volume's turned off, in black-and-white
from a room's corner, ashtrays filling with

what her lungs cannot, in the end, absorb.
Her eyes are bleary, sunk in, with dark rings,
tender from life's beating. Did such a place
exist? I imagine huge banyan trees
encircling the nearby swamp, their ropes
dragging the whole world down into jungle;
screams of monkeys at dusk, and the knowledge
that when they were quieted, danger lurked;
the hopelessness of learning Beethoven
in a small Cuban town, her father's cigarette
decomposing to cinder while she played.
There was a patio; a fountain tinkled.
She has his eyes, dark and handsome and beaten.
Miami's highways purr outside somewhere,
like unseen predators hunting the dark.
As she smokes, the TV making its ghosts
dance on her linoleum floor, I see
again the resemblance. I see her breathe,
inhaling memories, becoming him.
Now, almost quiet, it is almost safe.

III. ANXIETY

It's 1969. I'm five. The man
is knocking. Green shag carpet like a lawn
of chemicals. My mother vacuums it.
I fear the television's cloudy eye.
The man is knocking at our door. Outside,
it's winter in New Jersey, confusing
what's dry, what's cold: the salt-stained street looks parched,
my mother's face looks sunburned. The man knocks;
he has a black briefcase, looks official.
She mutters to herself, like we're in church.
Outside, the winter day seems tilted in the small
suburban windows of our house, a "ranch"
that lacks the cattle and the horses of

my father's fabled Cuban past. He knocks.
My father combs his hair so carefully
it's like he's trying to tell me something.
The vacuum cleaner whines with righteous rage,
soft pings of detritus consumed oddly
satisfying. Meanwhile, the knocking stops.
My mother studies lamp shades, curtains, me,
the vacuum cleaner whining at her feet.
She bites her lower lip, alone with us,
alone with winter's tilted, cold, dry days;
the kitchen sparkles with her loneliness,
as if being seen through a film of tears.
I realize I fear he won't come back,
that we can never return home again.

Advanced Placement

Señora Haines is blond and has big tits,
the reason mostly guys enroll. We get

to pick our Spanish names: I choose Raúl.
My girlfriend Sally is Pilar. The school

reminds me of the plastic packaging
my dad brings home from work, tubes and weird things

American Can says will make life better.
"You don't pronounce the 'h'"—and so we wonder

exactly what to call our teacher. Down
the hall, the polished floors emit a sound

silent as gleaming, almost like desire.
I realize I don't love Sally. "Liar,"

she calls me when I grope at her flat chest
under the bleachers, while the others blast

baseballs into the infinite white sky.
We settle on just plain "Señora." "Y

is I GRIEGA," she writes in sloped script,
the Spanish painted on her full red lips

a shade lighter than what my tía wears,
the one who drinks and teaches me to swear:

"Pendejo. Hijo de puta. Cabrón."
I mouth the words, but lack her venom.

"You never learn, you too soft from this place,"
she garbles her English, pinching my face.

She's right. I only took this class to get
an A. Pilar stares past me. My ears hurt.

Elegy for a Revolution

You, ghost of Cuba, vestige of a dream,
what makes me pity you? Your stout cigar
now trembles in your scaly hands, your beard
is thin and gray like my abuela's hair.
Strange that I preferred you when you were gruff
and threatening, almost sexy in
those olive-green fatigues, thundering
your condemnations of America.
You were huge like my father, furious.
One Christmas, I asked Santa Claus for Cuba,
as if the island were a plaything that
a spoiled child could own; years later, still
bereft, I wrote to you directly, begged
for your forgiveness, begged to be rescued
like my Tía Marta was, who eloped
one starless night with a Puerto Rican guard
stationed at the base in Guantánamo.
I wanted freedom, yet you proved as cruel
as any Latin lover, promising
your heart, but giving only loyalty.
You were the first man I ever loved, but
your arranged marriage to that ugly hag
of your own hubris was the end of us.
You, ghost of Cuba, now your insides rot.
Some say that you're dead already, but not
to me, your Yankee whore, your last great hope,
your forsaken joy, your sworn enemy—
I pity you and your outrageous dream.

Patriotic Anthem for a Lost Homeland

on the fiftieth anniversary of the Communist revolution in Cuba

It is the way of revolutions: worlds
turned upside down, but only until words

begin again to redefine what was
as what went wrong. O Cuba, did you wash

away all injustice, make greed extinct?
Has capitalism gone to the brink

of excess you condemned so forcefully?
No revolution honors memory,

so you will once again deny my faith,
the scar on my grandfather's sun-worn face,

and even your own people's successes.
It is the way of revolution: less

will be retold as more, lies will be truth,
and fifty years from now, there will be proof

that neither one of us was right. O Cuba,
admit your failures, say we too are human,

say it, that all of us are joined in that
same hope. The revolution in my heart

keeps mixing oxygen with blood, despair
with passion. Someday, I will breathe the air

of your green mountains. Words will fill my head,
and what I say will have been almost dead

for fifty years. I will dream, "Cuba, have you
missed me?" "O Cuba," I will vow, "I love you."

Resort

for my father

I wonder if his memories omit
the same things that we don't see here. He stares
out at the view, which is as tropical
as it is trite. The grounds are orderly,
the jacaranda are in bloom. No one
is poor. Like lions caged too long, the waves
loll lazily along the beach. He stares
out at the bright horizon, lost in thought.
I wonder if his memories might hurt.
Tonight, beneath a moon as clear and plain
as need, we'll drink banana daiquiris.
He'll ask the mariachi band to play
a Cuban song, which they'll almost get right.
But in the morning, he must realize,
we'll still awaken here. Same sun, same sea,
same staring out involuntarily:
the simulation, if more dream than real,
is close enough. The birds-of-paradise,
though mute and flightless, still seem nearly free.

New Jersey, the Garden State

"A state of mind," my grandfather would say,
the sun as fierce as Mr. Cossimo's
critiques of everything, from his wife's sauce
to Senator Bill Bradley. Usually,
we talked about his garden, where he grew
tomatoes, Swiss chard, peppers, cucumbers,
and white eggplant he said were better than
the Cossimos'. "A state of mind, grandson."
He talked in quiet tones, as if suspicious
of his gigantic dahlias, which were
as tall as I was, leaning in from beds
he tended just as faithfully. "A state
of mind," I said to myself, mimicking
his resignation to such forces I
could never understand—like those that caused
the cucumbers to grow, they were, like God,
or like whatever kept my grandmother's
bouffant hairdo from collapse, powerful
and yet mysterious. He himself was bald,
like Mr. Cossimo, but not as fat,
which made me sometimes wonder whether that
was really why he thought his eggplants were
superior, and why they disagreed
on politics, religion, and the Mets.
"The Lord is everywhere," he'd say,
"so why they need to put Him in the laws?"
Lunchtime we sat outside, splayed in lawn chairs,
him with his wine and me with my Kool-Aid.
We'd admire the huge dahlias; I'd look
for God in the tomatoes. "State of mind,"
he murmured to himself, dozing. Inside,
my grandmother and my two great-aunts cooked
a feast for the whole family, black pots

releasing steam at intervals as if
divulging the forbidden love affairs
of those who stirred them ever warily,
while God kept watch like in Calabria.
That kitchen was too small for all those large
Italian women, whose torpedo breasts
would smother me as they leaned over us
to serve. With darkness falling, baseball on
the radio, I knew they'd be back soon.
The headlights washed the house in ghostly white;
bugs' shadows flitted magnified against
the blank expanse of the shut garage door.
"A state of mind," I told my parents when
they questioned me about my day. I held
a shopping bag on my sunburned lap,
heavy with fragrant, ripe tomatoes. "God,"
I told them, crying, "He is everywhere."

Rio Grande

I have a drug cartel inside my heart,
and they're killing innocent bystanders,
like those parrots in Frida Kahlo's art
and the gods of the Aztec calendar.

Who wouldn't think of leaving this desert
where zero was invented? Millions now
look to Texas and the Spanish defeat,
remembering the goddamn Alamo

as if they had nothing to lose. Across
the border in my decrepit hometown
the *viejitas* are skeletons dressed
in black, pure mourning: another son drowns

in this great test of our humanity.
We never learned to swim in bitterness;
to us, the river's water's flow is free.
We're all addicted to some form of grace,

the Spanish translation of which is pain.
Great River, cleanse us of sin, carry us
like corpuscles in the deepest of veins.
Heroin's heroism, maze of maize:

America is paved in gold, they say.
I squint at the distance, but what I see
is haze. Guns fire, executing the day;
my dreams make the crossing to memory.

Fish Story

Some lies we can't help but forgive: the one
that got away, the unaccounted-for
ten pounds, where you were, father, on those days
you missed the baseball game or the class trip.

I'd say you were on business in Taiwan,
invent a secret mission somewhere spies
lived their unfaithful lives. I watched your face
at dinnertime, but you were perfect in

your alias, your smile inscrutable,
your weariness believable, your eyes
averted. Following your lead, I told
you everything was fine, my heart like tin,

my head like wood. The kitchen light was dull;
even the dog seemed fake, wagging his tail
not joyfully, but out of need unfilled.
One night, you said you'd take me to the lake

to go fishing. Morning came so on time
it seemed like just another plot. We sailed
on placid water, lines plumbing the depths,
the immensity of what we might hook

impossible to say. Some commit crimes,
while other men tell lies we could forgive:
The fish that broke the rod, the wish that leapt
just out of reach, the one that got away.

Times Square

Six stories tall, displaying perfect abs,
he floats above the yellow taxicabs:

Apollo, clad in underwear. It was
to us nothing less than miraculous,

two kids from Bergen County thinking we
were lost, amid the throngs impossibly

converging there. But we were never more
assuredly *someplace*, where Broadway bore

down brilliantly from Central Park, as if
it were a river not yet overfished,

still full of dreams and possibilities.
Still teenagers, we'd purchased fake IDs—

ironic, now, in retrospect. We'd kissed
before, but no one ever witnessed it:

here, we'd have the world's attention! Marquees
throbbed rhythmically with all the urgency

of heartbeats, an odd lady cursed and sang;
some Puerto Rican dudes were breakdancing

around a huge boom box's thundering.
The pigeons' iridescent spiraling

marked the center of the whole universe—
while everywhere, America in force,

the countless flags at once hubris and grace.
He leaned toward me, tilting up his young face,

eyes closed in the crowd's get-on-with-it embrace.

Calendar

I threw out 1998 today.
What had I hoped for then, what days were marked?
My grandfather was dead that year, by March.
We mourned him in the cemetery's gray,

wishing we had some lost time with him back.
"You can't hold on to memories," he'd say,
his lungs half-gone, his heart long since betrayed.
He kept a yellowing almanac

on some shelves near his bed. Some fishing lures,
and toy soldiers and photographs—bright days
that he somehow kept on living, the phase
of the black moon each week less of a cure.

Best planting days, lost anniversaries—
what do we know? Thrown open in the trash
those since-forgotten months, the perfect halves
of equinox, the year's early first freeze.

The Thief

The poet is a thief, and nothing more.
I started relatively small: I stole
a glance at you at first, and later on,

I stole a moment in your quiet gaze.
Before too long, I started stealing more.
I stole an image from your library,

a standard form that could belong to me
as much as anyone. The poet is
a thief, and nothing more. I stole your heart,

and spilled a bit of it as I rushed out
the door; I stole a definition of
what some might say is poetry itself.

The poet is a thief, an awful bore.
I started getting more audacious. Steeled
to anyone but you, I took what things

I could. I stuffed my pockets with your shame,
I robbed you of your self-esteem. I stole
the smoke from your lit cigarette. I stole

your first uncertain kiss, I stole whole lives
that neither one of us could ever live.
I stole a car, I stole policemen too,

I even stole your reputation. Soon,
I stole so much I couldn't look at you.
I spilled some stolen tears; I spilled my guts,

but even my confession seemed untrue.
I'd stolen that pathetic gesture too.
The poet is a thief, a whore. I stole

some time with you while you still tried to write.
I knew what you were doing: stealing night,
unlocking secrets, taking all you could.

A common thief and nothing more: you thought
I pitied you. Instead, I saw the petty thief
that you are too, who almost stole the world.

Batteries Not Included

I left out the part where I told a lie.
Forgot to mention my inveterate
invisibility. You see, my sky
is falling but I can't seem to escape

unfortunate conclusions. What I said
makes little difference. It was self-defense.
It was 8:30 in the morning. Kids
remind me of confetti, in a sense—

they seem to cover playgrounds having swirled
down from above. I left the hard part out.
He made me think I was a little girl,
invisible. Inconclusive Boy Scout,

I never solved the riddle, never came
to know who did this. The psychiatrist:
"An unremarkable account of pain."
And still I wince every time I'm kissed,

look up at the sky because I fear I might
be stricken down by God knows what. I still
don't know the truth. I still cry at the sight
of confetti, and I hate grape popsicles.

I left out the part where the world tells lies
about its own repeating beauty. See
the sky, observe the sun as it defies
our words to describe its enormity;

remember we are nothing here. We hurt
so we can have a reason to forgive.
I see his fingernails, his pinstriped suit.
I lie to my own heart, can't help but live.

Kids' Games

1. PIN THE TAIL ON THE DONKEY

Your birthday party, 1969.
Some laughing parents, all drinking red wine.
Piñata dangling, bulging with promised sweets.
Flimsy cardboard gamepiece. My heart's loud beats
while I am blindfolded. A woman's hands
spin me in perfumed blackness. I extend
my arm toward that awkward ass,
a spectacle of need and helplessness.

2. SMEAR THE QUEER

A spectacle of need and helplessness:
I'm fourteen years old, and the way I dress
must make it obvious, if not to me.
The beatings seem to happen tenderly,
almost without force. I know I'll see them
later, in class or the gymnasium.
Just like Jesus does in church when I pray,
they won't acknowledge me; they'll look away.

3. MONKEY IN THE MIDDLE

They won't acknowledge me. They'll look away
when I approach. I must have overplayed
my hand. I stand there silently between
them. They converse as if through a dark screen.
I will never forgive myself for that.
It's just me, myself, and my constant guilt.
It's late, and anyway, I've always hated
parties—birthdays shouldn't be celebrated.

Heart Grow Fonder

for Eve

The leg bone's connected to the shin bone.
An apple a day keeps the doctor away.
A little voice inside me said, "Beware."

A tumor big as a grapefruit killed her.
Tamoxifen, oxycodone, Bengay.
The breastbone's connected to the rib bone.

Like a patient etherized, I can't say
what evening looks like, but I feel alone.
A little voice inside me said, "Unfair."

"My brain's a sieve," she'd say. We mourned her hair.
She'd get lost on the way to San Jose.
The rib bone's connected to the back bone.

I plunged my heart in San Francisco bay.
A scar across her chest: one breast was gone.
A little voice inside me said, "I'm scared."

Some final pleasures: slices of ripe pear,
massages strangely not unlike foreplay.
The back bone's connected to the neck bone.

Old voicemails from her that I still replay.
"Physician, heal thyself," sweetly intones
the little voice inside me I can't bear.

We'd read together almost every day.
After great pain, a formal feeling comes—
the neck bone's connected to the head bone.
A little voice inside me says, "Beware."

Trees

What's left to write about but trees? These here
for instance, photosynthesizing words
from sun and air, their leaves the way we hear
whatever wind might have to say. I heard

your name again, and it still hurt. What's left
to write about but you? We sat beneath
these trees, and I remember how you laughed
at me for staring at you while you breathed,

as if I could discern what lived in you
that seemed to animate my soul. What's left
to write about if not the soul, the few
diminishing, delirious last gifts

of you, your words, your sighs, your laugh. These stars
cannot remember anything, and yet
they do, by keeping their particular
arrangement well beyond the trees, the wet

grass wet as it once was back then. I'll write
about these trees tonight, about fireflies,
about sitting with you here as daylight
faded, about our need to tell these lies:

"I love you," said so particularly
that even I believed you; the soul,
though not human, does not exist in trees;
there's nothing left to write about. I still

remember you that way, the rustling
of leaves above us saying something new,
in songs that only trees know how to sing.
Initials carved in bark: "RC + U,"

because you said you wouldn't ever be
immortalized. And yet we live to be called
to such a place as this; we write these trees,
whose names are carved, like yours, upon my soul.

Promnesia

I have memories of places I have
never visited: a worn, stained oak table
in southern Spain where I write mournful poems
about strange places never visited;

a beach like any other beach except
somehow I know I'm in Cuba; a town,
New Hampshire maybe, with a cemetery
of tombstones from the eighteenth century;

or China, where a billion people live
but don't remember me, though I'm quite sure
I lost my way among them on a rural road.
It is enough, I suppose, just to wish

I had been there, where I might have been delighted
by the child I never had, or the sun's
illumination of that question I
have always longed to ask myself. I write

the line that's ever just eluded me;
I write about the photograph I lost
of just the two of us, happy, the way
we once were. I write about the same rain

that falls again, and how it always seems
disgruntled; books I read by the gray light
are filled with sentences no doubt I've read
before. I want to love you, too—but think

about these gardens I don't know, about
the hearts of other creatures I could swear
I studied in a library that seems
like elsewhere, full of so much forgetting.

The Reading

In a clearing bounded by Philosophy
and Self-Help, twenty folding chairs stood fast
in little lines lean as a poem. Most
were empty still, like possibilities
that might yet be considered. Patiently,
a few dignified older ladies sat,
and in the back, scowling, the requisite
unbalanced but still harmless refugee
of the city's more insensitive streets.
Pathetic, if not insignificant
it seemed, as the cash registers up front
scanned tell-alls of gay stars who once were straight
and novels coding what we're told we seek.
A pair of college students drifted in,
their composition notebooks and pale skin
blank, ready to be written on. None spoke
until one of the bored store managers
appeared and gave the introduction. Brief
applause. Then, just as she began to read,
you took my hand, to meet the universe.

II.

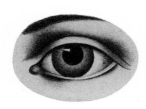

ALTERNATIVE

MEDICINE

Hospital Song

Someone is dying alone in the night.
The hospital hums like a consciousness.
I see their faces where others see blight.

The doctors make their rounds like satellites,
impossible to fathom distances.
Someone is dying alone under lights,

deficient in some electrolyte.
A mother gives birth: life replenishes.
I see pain in her face where others see fright.

A woman with breast cancer seems to be right
when she refuses our assurances
that we won't let her die alone tonight;

I see her face when I imagine flight,
when I dream of respite. Life punishes
us, faces searching ours for that lost light

which we cannot restore, try as we might.
The nurses' white sneakers say penances,
contrite as someone dying in the night.

As quiet as mercy, the morning's rites
begin. Over an old man's grievances,
his face contorted in the early light,

an aide serenely tends to him, her slight
black figure fleeting, yet all hopefulness—
her face the face of others who see light,
like someone dying at peace in the night.

Faith Healing

The tiny silver crucifix she wore
enacted what it seemed we did to her.

She rested in the bed, not at peace yet,
she said, but trying to forgive. The dead

moved quietly around the room, unseen:
last week, a man with liver cancer keened

where she did now, before he passed; and then
another woman whose lymphoma drenched

her in cold sweats, her lymph nodes thick and massed
wherever I had pressed. "Dear Lord," I said,

attempting what I thought was prayer, "—Lord,
forgive me for not healing them." Unsaid,

the words of her forgiveness came to me
like kindness, like a sudden memory.

The tiny crucifix refused to bleed;
instead, it shone there like a misplaced need,

a way to understand the blameless night.
Adjusting my ophthalmoscope's light,

I peered inside her, seeking what we may
of pain. I saw what she had tried to say:

the pulse of blood, the silence of my heart;
forgiveness, not impossible, but hard.

Iatrogenic

You say, "I do this to myself." Outside,
my other patients wait. Maybe snow falls;
we're all just waiting for our deaths to come,
we're all just hoping it won't hurt too much.
You say, "It makes it seem less lonely here."
I study them, as if the deep red cuts
were only wounds, as if they didn't hurt
so much. The way you hold your upturned arms,
the cuts seem aimed at your unshaven face.
Outside, my other patients wait their turns.
I run gloved fingertips along their course,
as if I could touch pain itself, as if
by touching pain I might alleviate
my own despair. You say, "It's snowing, Doc."
The snow, instead of howling, soundlessly
comes down. I think you think it's beautiful;
I say, "This isn't all about the snow,
is it?" The way you hold your upturned arms,
I think about embracing you, but don't.
I think, "We do this to ourselves." I think
the falling snow explains itself to us,
blinding, faceless, and so deeply wounding.

The Third Step in Obtaining an Arterial Blood Gas

First, gather your equipment: squares of gauze,
iodine swab, needle (23-gauge),
and don't forget the cup of ice you need
to send it to the lab. Next, find the pulse
(did I forget to mention sterile gloves?)
between your index and third fingers where
you need to make your stick. Press hard enough,
obliterating it for just a beat
or two, imagining the artery—
release the pressure gently as you bend
back the patient's wrist. See the artery
beneath the skin, and as you aim, don't think,
this part's the hardest part, don't think about
the pain, just focus on the flash of red
that means you're in. Then hold it steady as
the plunger moves invisibly, like God
or the force of your will is moving it—
the blood draws itself, pretty fucking cool,
huh? Just like magic, right—but it's really not.
Now practice one on that gorked CVA
we just admitted. She won't feel a thing.

After the Floods

The doctors had to let the patients die.
The hospital, more obviously drowning—
instead of woe, it was filthy floodwaters—
had no place left to keep its data dry.

Imagine: charts float through a door, whole lives
adrift upon an ink-black tide. They had
to let the patients die, because the world
itself was in congestive failure. Leaves,

a cardboard box, a crumpled silk brassiere:
the ward is humbled by the detritus
of those it sheltered once. The doctors fled,
but helped the wordless patients die before

the waters rose too high, their faces moist,
their bedclothes billowing, their bodies light,
finally, done with the toils of the flesh.
The doctors gave their patients one last choice:

To die with dignity or in the brine
of anonymity. I hope they held
their listless, wasted hands, as black and cold
arrived each death the doctors' medicine

invited down. When they were done, the day
was somehow even quieter. A gun
was fired in the distance, then flamed the sun.
The doctors had to help their patients die.

For All the Freaks of the World

after Mary Campbell

A friend of mine once wrote a poem for Buttons,
then famous as the world's smallest horse.
I felt sorry for her, my friend I mean,
because all she could see was the irony,
the confinement of such a spectacle
in such a pitifully small stall.

Then there was Mister Pinky, the world's smallest dog:
five inches tall, dressed in a pink tux
complete with tiny bow tie
and a dapper pink fedora.
I was shocked to learn he's really a she.
I read about it in the newspaper.

I went to a conference once
and met a woman who was once a man.
She had severe liver failure, and wanted
to write a poem about her illness.
She said the hospital made her crazy.
I tried to help her. I'm not sure if I did.

I looked in the mirror this morning
and stared at my pitifully thinning hair.
When I was in college, a girl who liked me
but didn't know I was gay
said I looked like George Michael.
We remember the weirdest things.

There's a couple of well-nourished queers
whose wedding announcement
appears in the Sunday paper
complete with a picture of them
in their white tuxes and white bow ties
feeding each other huge mouthfuls of cake.

A friend of mine, who is a nearsighted poet,
tells me her girlfriend is leaving her.
She can't earn a decent living wage
teaching composition at MIT.
Someone should write a poem about
the billions her students will make cloning genes
and curing cancer, or liver failure.

I read in the newspaper once
about some poor sheep named Dolly
who was made to give birth to her own clone.
They looked alike. I thought it was ironic,
because who can tell the difference
between most sheep anyway?

When I was a student
at Harvard Medical School,
I worked in an immunology lab
that was run by a Holocaust survivor's son.
The research involved harvesting eyes
from genetically mutant, hairless mice.
I can't remember much else.

Once, I tried to help a homeless man in the street.
"I'm a doctor," I said.
His breath stank of vomit,
and one eye was white like glue.
His belly was swollen from liver failure.
He said I had hands like a woman's.

Sometimes I wish I could see Buttons
in her pitiful little stall.
After, I'd eat a corn dog and a fried Twinkie,
then climb a hill to be alone
with the wind in my remaining hair
to write a poem for all the freaks of the world.

Pharmacopeia for the New Millennium

1. AMPLIA

For the aversion of consequences,
specifically of overeating. Take
ten tablets with a bottle of red wine,
three Big Macs, cold leftover lasagna,
and one pint of cookie dough ice cream.
Adverse reactions include surliness,
increased drowsiness while watching TV,
and in men, increased morning drowsiness
or an erection that won't go away
while watching TV. Call your doctor if
you experience the need to sue for
a raging case of diabetes or
heart disease, which is really no one's fault.

2. HERONIL

Highly effective for the absence of
inspiring leaders. May also be prescribed
for the treatment of illegitimate
elections, lack or loss of civil rights,
and disgust with supreme judicial courts.
Side effects include forgetfulness, nice
dreams, extreme cynicism, and some doubts
about the threat posed by terrorism.
To be taken immediately, if
clean drinking water is available.
WARNING: Women should avoid handling
broken or damaged tablets, for reasons
that are obvious. Call your doctor if
you realize he is a senator
who might become the next president, and
who has made millions of dollars from
shady corporate health care boondoggles,

while millions of Americans, many of whom
will vote for him, cannot afford this drug.

3. CALDONIX

In large clinical trials, has been shown
to decrease awareness of increasing
ambient temperatures. Mechanism
of action is poorly understood, but
may be related to lower threshold
for cranking up the AC. Adverse events
can be debated endlessly while we
measure the rate at which polar ice caps
melt. Rising sea levels may or may not
be related. Nonbiased consultants'
reports suggest that more Americans
worry about Pluto's planetary
status than the certain disappearance
of the island nations of Tuvalu
and the Maldives. May also interact
with other new drugs like Amplia and
Heronil, causing a rise in serum
drug levels and neurotoxicity.
Call your doctor if you have no one else
to call, or if you missed the episode
of *Survivor: Vanuatu* in which
Lars votes Kim off after calling her a bitch.

4. WIKIPOR

Used to control delusions of control,
democratic knowledge-sharing, and all
other false hopes engendered by too much
surfing on the Internet. May cause hives
if taken while downloading music files
illegally or checking out porn sites.

Induce vomiting immediately
if ingested accidentally. Call
your doctor if you want a computer
but can't afford one, for a prescription
for a generic sedative instead.

5. EMPATHASE

Indicated for the reduction of
despair associated with the loss
of compassion. Hopeless romantics and
hand-wringing, bleeding-heart liberals may
also see some improvement with chronic
use. May be habit forming. Maybe not.
May be taken on a full stomach if
not impoverished. May heighten certain
spiritual impulses, while others
may be diminished. May cause the pooled blood
of an adulteress condemned to death by
stoning to look like the Virgin Mary.
May cause black men and homosexuals
to be mistaken for our brothers. Call
your doctor now to get your free sample
and find out if treatment is right for you.

Recent Past Events

It wasn't so miraculous back then.
Some said we had their blood on our prim hands.
We were ashamed of our good appetites.
We marched together in gay pride parades.
We feared their blood. We prayed for it to end.
We learned the names of lands in Africa:
Botswana, Ghana, Tanzania, Chad.
We adopted universal precautions.
We prayed for it to end. We feared their blood.
We were afraid to call our parents who
we knew would think the worst. We learned to speak
in acronyms. We watched two women kiss
on television late one night. We cried.
We handed out free condoms in the Fens.
Remember when it seemed miraculous
that most of our close friends weren't dead? We feared
their blood. We were ashamed. We went on trips
to Africa. We saw a leopard kill
an antelope, we saw the vast red dunes
Namibia is famous for. We cried
at patients' funerals. We handed out
clean needles in the Fens. We feared their blood.
We touched each other carefully at night,
remembered when it felt miraculous.
Remember when his cheekbones didn't jut out
so much? We had their blood on our clean hands.
We were ashamed of living while they died.
We cooked for friends. We prayed for it to end.
We traveled to Peru, New Zealand, France.
We bungee-jumped from cliffs, we sipped red wine,
we shopped for clothes that fit us well. We watched
the president announce more funds. We cried.
We were ashamed of our good appetites.

We watched two women kiss outside the door
of our favorite Chinese restaurant.
We talked about adopting kids. We feared
what people thought of us. We bought a house.
We painted the back bedroom red like blood.
We gave less money to the charities.
We found a nice church that accepted us.
The stained glass windows seemed miraculous.
We ate our dinner. We remembered how
we feared their blood, and how we prayed for it
to end. And how it never really did.

Alternative Medicine

Wednesday afternoon HIV clinic

I. ADVERSE REACTION

"Pray for me," she asks, her head covered in
a polyester scarf. She doesn't hide
herself for shame; she's lost her hair. We think
it was the AZT. She says that through
the walls of all her suffering, she thinks
she hears God's distant voice when her young son
reads from his new storybook. She's so proud
he's learning English. "Pray for him," she asks
before she leaves, "that he may have enough
to bury me in a fine new white dress!"

II. FAILURE TO THRIVE

He weighs less than ninety pounds. Years ago,
he was a bodybuilder. Muscular
and tanned, he looks like someone else back then,
the photograph he shows me faded now.
"You know, even my cock has shriveled up,"
he says. "No one would want to fuck me now."
He undresses very slowly; I count
his ribs while he fumbles with the blue gown.
When I touch him, he avoids my eyes, stares
up at the blank ceiling instead, and cries.

III. LEUKOPENIA

I see him sometimes when I'm walking home.
He holds his children's hands, refuses to
acknowledge me. I know his viral load,
his T cell count, his medication list,
as if these data somehow pinpoint him.

Enveloped in the park's expanse of snow,
his two small children bobbing next to him
like life preservers, I remember that
he's leukopenic. Snow begins to fall
again, innumerable tiny white flakes.

IV. ADVANCED DIRECTIVES

The rescue regimen is failing too.
He lives alone in an AIDS SRO,
once had two little shih-tzu mixes he
was forced to give up—the neighbors complained
about the barking. Not depressed, he says.
Not suicidal. Still taking his meds.
He watches Oprah, gets a hot lunch daily.
I write the orders in his chart. He says
it's funny, since his mother always said
she wished he'd never been born anyway.

V. CARDIOMYOPATHY

He can't tie his shoes anymore because
his feet are so swollen. Denies chest pain
but says his heart aches, whatever that means.
Ejection fraction less than thirty now.
Strange that it keeps progressing, since the meds
have kept his virus undetectable.
He says he doesn't drink, is sober now
for fifteen years. Assessing the edema,
I leave the imprint of my fingertips
anywhere I press down on his taut skin.

VI. RESISTANCE

I think she must be missing doses, since
she hasn't yet disclosed her status to
her husband, who she fears will leave her—or
worse, if he finds out she's positive now.
Good question—he probably exposed her,
but that's not the point. Here's her genotype:
clean, no resistance mutations at all.
Her virus is wild-type, and so she should
suppress on her twice-a-day regimen.
Either that, or she's just not taking it.

VII. IVDU

 "I envy you," he says. "You got it all
figured." I stare at the computer screen.
"IVDU. That means I'm on dope, right?
Just an addict, right?" Silently, I type.
"You got to write me a prescription, man.
IVDU? A-I-D-S. That's AIDS.
Can't you just be happy I'm gonna die
and give me my damn prescription?" I try
to hate him, but write "Percocet" instead.
"Now, that didn't hurt much, did it?" he asks.

VIII. UNIVERSAL PRECAUTIONS

You tell me that like me you must wear gloves
at work, restoring precious paintings at
the MFA. Imagining you bent
intently over some scarred masterwork,
I wonder whether your light touch might heal,
but in another sense: I must protect
us all should suddenly you bleed, while you
expose us to the curious infection
of what is possible to know by life's
wounds. Even through my gloves, your skin feels warm.

IX. OPPORTUNISTIC INFECTION

She tells me that her dream involved a cliff—
no, mountain—that she climbed until she reached
its peak. From there, she saw a pristine view:
unending valleys, white-gray glaciers, snow.
The air was thin and she could hardly breathe.
She suddenly began to cough, and blood
poured out of her like song. But in the dream,
she didn't have tuberculosis yet;
she's sure she was infected with a lie,
and inside her, it was the dream that died.

X. ALTERNATIVE MEDICINE

I won't take antiretrovirals, don't
eat processed foods, and remain celibate.
I will take echinacea for a cold—
I wish all medicines came from the earth
and not some toxic lab where they kill rats
with chemicals they claim "treat" HIV.
I exercise six times a week, and pray
to my own God. I believe that someday
we'll find the cure, and I'll be here to say
that one of us survived to celebrate.

Band of Gold

You told me "the lesser-known lesbians"
like Willa Cather and Alice Toklas
who died unremarkable, quiet deaths
never interested you. After all,
who wouldn't drink or pine themselves into
oblivion alone like that, unloved?
The only reason you were homeless was
because you beat up your brother Leon
after he called you a dyke and your folks
threw you out. You painted your nails pink
while you listened to Freda Payne belt out
"Band of Gold" over and over again.
You said she really knew what she was
talking about, because your girlfriend
left you when she found out you had cancer
and it hurt in exactly the same way.
You said your guess was she was probably
queer too, but since it was the seventies
you couldn't sing about another woman
breaking your heart like that. I was there
when you told the surgeon, sure he could
cut them off, but how would he like it if
someone cut off his cock? After you died
alone in your room one night, your mother
showed up with some hash brownies she'd baked you,
which were too sweet and didn't get us high.
The solarium felt like the inside
of emptiness, bright and airless and hot.
She told me that Leon had moved out, and
Freda Payne was a pretty black woman
who could pass for white and whose sister
was a back-up singer for the Supremes.
She had a film career that not many

people know about because of that
goddamn song, that whenever you hear it
you understand, whatever love might be,
it abandons us all us, mercilessly.

Primary Care

You, body, bleed, you stink, you interrupt
with plaintive sounds as if we didn't know
you suffer. Dressed in youth, you dazzle me
with your perfection, body: your two knees,
two eyes, two nipples, your fraught symmetries.
O body, even as you age you sing,
you are tender in certain places, you
believe you could be dying. Body, please,
repair yourself once more, bleed and stink,
decay again until, beneath your fragile skin,
I see the outlines of the soul you shield.
You, body, you will come again to me,
I see you naked in the shower, in
the mirror, realize that somehow you
must never die. O body, you are us,
all any of us have when we are lost.
You are immodest; you are honesty.
I see how careful you are when you bleed,
and when you stink it is god's grief we smell.
You, body, weep, you think, you scar as if
to show us our own history, as if
we didn't know. Body bleed, body stink,
remind us that we suffer, yes, remind
us that we must, or else we never lived.

Nude

I enter unexpectedly, and see
your hair cascading white-and-gray in loose,
long tresses down the full length of your back.
The nurse is bathing you in honeyed light,
when sunrise in the hospital makes all
seem gorgeous, even the gleaming bedpan,
even the scuffed but bright linoleum,
even the faces peering into death.
Your heart is failing, yet you have the strength
to turn, your breasts still the world's nourishment,
your eyes, though I have diagnosed in them
thick cataracts, alight again with youth's
demure, coquettish indignation. "Please,
excuse me Doctor, I am indisposed!"
For just a moment, as you pull the sheet
to safeguard your imperiled modesty—
your operatic thighs, your blatant hips,
your ruined neck with its distended veins—
I think you are like Goya's ageless nude,
eternal beckoning of human form,
inviolable, innocent, a gift
that both of us acknowledge, knowing that
such love is too sweet ever to be shared.

Not Untrue

Midnight, and he was asking for the score.
He was at a ball game, alive again—
not alone in the hospital, not scared
of dying like this with his mind half-gone.

I watched the clock, which sometimes could seem not
indifferent—sometimes, its face could seem kind—
but the second hand twitched like an insect,
reminding me that there's never more time.

His oxygen hissed, as if it could tell
secrets. The window previewed what was next:
nothing I could see, a perpetual
black emptiness. The nurse quietly knocked;

she grimaced wanly as she smoothed his sheets,
adjusted his IV, and left. He glared
at me, confused again. His voice was weak:
"Your goddamn mother never really cared."

Midnight still, the clock relentlessly read,
beneath which he seemed even smaller now.
"It's 3 to 1, bottom of the ninth, Dad."
Though I didn't know his name, it somehow

seemed forgivable to hold his chapped hand.
"She loved you, Dad. You know she always did."
I'm still not sure if he could understand,
but who can fault me, even if I lied.

On the Wards

I pass you in a hurry, on my way
to where another woman who I know
is dying of a stroke that in the end
is nothing worse than what is killing you.
Same gurney, same bruised arms and mute IV—
you wait for what might be a final test.
It's something in the way you look at me
that makes me realize you have your own
mistakes you think you're paying for, your own
ungrateful kids, your own unspeakable
pain. Yet you look at me, still desperate
for just another human being to
look kindly back at you, to recognize
in you the end is not far off, is not
so unimaginable. Years ago
I watched a patient of mine say goodbye
to life. She was alone like you, alone
like me, she was in agony. She looked
at me, and I, afraid to be the last
thing here on earth she saw, twisted my head
to look away. I almost do the same
to you, afraid you might imagine me
as later you lie dying, but I don't.
Instead, I look at you remorselessly,
the way I hope that someday I am seen,
the way each one deserves to be imagined,
if not restored to health, then spared this grief.

Without My White Coat

I'm not a real doc without my white coat.
I could be anyone: this sullen girl,
some homeless person crying to himself,
that addict who thinks he's got HIV.

I could be anyone: this sullen girl
who studies the ink stain on my white coat,
that addict who thinks he gave HIV
to his boyfriend, who sits in my waiting room.

He studies the ink stain on my white coat.
I wonder if he feels dirty, too.
His boyfriend, who sits in my waiting room,
looked up at me hopefully. I regret

my wondering; I feel dirty, too,
a brown-skinned imposter in my white coat.
"Look up," I say unhopefully, regret
the burning light I shine in his dark eyes;

a brown-skinned imposter in a white coat,
I'm half-surprised he follows my commands.
The burning light I shine in his dark eyes
constricts his pupils. When his tears well up,

I'm not surprised: he follows the commands
of human need. My white coat keeps me clean
and strict before my pupil. His tears well up
as carefully I draw his speechless blood.

Of human need, my white coat keeps me clean,
revealing very little of myself.
Carefully, speechlessly, I draw his blood:
a picture of the unseen soul, perhaps.

Revealing very little of myself,
my white coat holds my shape. Stands for something—
a picture of the unseen soul, perhaps.
Perhaps it is the ghost of who I was.

My white coat holds my shape, stands for something
universal—love, healing, peace. I am,
perhaps, a ghost of something that once was.
I wish I could be better than I am.

Universal love, healing peace: I am
the homeless person crying to himself,
wishing I could be better than I am.
I'm not a real doc without my white coat.

Health

While jogging on the treadmill at the gym,
that exercise in getting nowhere fast,
I realized we need a health pandemic.
Obesity writ large no more, Alzheimer's
forgotten, we could live carefree again.
We'd chant the painted shaman's sweaty oaths,
we'd kiss the awful relics of the saints,
we'd sip the bitter tea from twisted roots,
we'd listen to our grandmothers' advice.
We'd understand the moonlight's whispering.
We'd exercise by making love outside,
and afterward, while thinking only of
how much we'd lived in just one moment's time,
forgive ourselves for wanting something more:
to praise the memory of long-lost need,
or not to live forever in a world
made painless by our incurable joy.

Why Doctors Write

A doctor writes an order in the chart.
A doctor writes prescriptions to be filled.
A doctor writes the patient's history
in order to record it in the chart.
A doctor writes because she must. She writes
prescriptions that to patients seem like cures.
A doctor writes the mystery of death
in stark abbreviations: DNR—
do not resuscitate—and DNI.
A doctor writes prescriptions for more pills.
A doctor writes because he must, because
he watched another patient die last night.
A doctor wrote an order in the chart:
DO NOT INTUBATE, which the nurse transcribed.
A doctor writes invisibly upon
a patient's chest, the stethoscope's black curl
like punctuation, breath like poetry
heard almost lovingly. A doctor writes
because she must, because she can't deny
the body speaks, and what it tries to say
is more than what's recorded in the chart.
A doctor writes because he can't prevent
the heart attack, because he can't stop death
no matter what new pills he might prescribe.
A doctor writes an order in the chart.
A doctor writes a poem that no one reads.
A doctor writes because he must, because
not one of us can stop the final cure.
A doctor writes because she tried to stop
but couldn't. Nurses question orders; night
falls mercilessly again. Doctors write
because they must, because the ICU
is like a dream we think we can decode.

A doctor writes a poem in the chart,
though none can read its invisible lines,
or understand the mystery of death.

Reforming Health Care

I try to think of what I'm thankful for.
Parade of misery comes through my door:

dysuria, depression, hemorrhoids,
a lung mass that proved to be carcinoid,

low back pain that I've tried to diagnose,
strange tingling sensations in the nose

that honestly I haven't. What I do
so often seems frankly contrary to

my vision of myself as healer, noble
if undervalued shepherd to the feeble.

I try to think of what I'm thankful for.
As I examine someone's painful sore,

I wonder if I'm thankful I'm not him.
Adderall, Oxycontin, Valium:

I wonder if I'm thankful that relief
might yet be possible, that in this life

there is suffering, yes, but there is peace.
The classic rash of lupus marks the face

the beautiful young woman I see next
has tried to cover with a scarf as best

she can. It's not shaped like a butterfly,
I see when she reveals it; when she cries,

I don't pretend it's sweet music, or bleed
from some wound I can't trade for hers. Instead,

I grasp at last what I'm still thankful for:
not the disease that lets me comfort her,

or my unexceptional abilities
however insufficient they might be,

but in the final absence of a cure,
the need in all of us for someone's care.

The Performance

Wish Bone the cancer clown came up
to BMT today. The kids
lined up in the solarium,
in two squat rows that looked just like
a dozen blighted eggs, bald heads
shining, the sun on them too bright
as if a miracle were near.
He started with some jokes: *What's black*
and white and red all over? Knock-
knock? Who's there? Anita. It's who?
I need a hug right now! They laughed
so hard that one of them, the girl
with no platelets, got a nosebleed.
He twisted up balloons to look
like dachshunds and giraffes, then some
odd shape I didn't recognize
which probably was a mistake
but Deb the nurse said could have been
the knot that formed inside her throat
as shamelessly we lapped it up.
The punch arrived, its blobs of pink
and green sherbet melting, like them
not long for this world. As we left
we grabbed some cookies, happy we
could savor what we knew, in spite
of what we hoped, was cruel joy.

III.

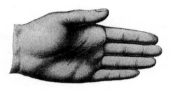

PLONK

Ode to the Lists in Front of Me

Ten things to do today.
Class list: six women's names.
Some illnesses I don't
yet have. A verse or two.
The colors we might paint
our bedroom. List of lists!
Today, I'd like to list
instead the sounds that drift
unbidden through the door:
the shrieking neighbors' kids,
the leaves conversing with
the wind, the song of birds
I wish I paid attention
to more often. List of lists:
The wind and leaves again,
not just a conversation
but litanies of truths,
the birdsong listing what
is beautiful. Your face
is beautiful, the way
it lists the places where
we've been, our arguments,
wrinkles enumerating joys,
eyebrows, freckles, nose,
your teeth, your eyes, your smile.
You who love lists, in your eyes
the lists you make for us:
The Costco list, the ten
world wonders we must see
before we die, the most
important rights we gained
when we could marry, the
master list of anniversaries

and birthdays we absolutely
must never forget, your top
three favorite colors, the ten
reasons you love me. I try
to make a list today:
these several women's names
might guard the secrets of
the universe, what the birds
say could save my dull life,
and in the conversation
of leaves and winds, the power
to open doors invisibly,
to teach unendingly
how we might yet survive.

LAX

"Don't talk to me, I'm driving." Palm trees sway
beneath a sky of airplanes, sky of blue.
I think we're lost, but don't know what to say.

Beneath a sky of airplanes, sky of blue
an enemy descended. Something frayed.
We pass another parking lot, asphalt gloom.

Don't talk to me—I'm praying as they sway,
reliving those twin towers, love and doom.
I'm sure we're lost. I hope my flight's delayed.

O sky of blue, beneath you we are few:
An endless movie set, an endless day,
Black, Muslim, homosexual, and Jew—

are they lost, those Mexicans who we say
must be illegal? We pass them by, dimmed in the blue-
gray haze of the car's exhaust. Palm trees sway,

reminding us to witness beauty's truth,
that place where minds end, where the longest day
begins again. We're lost, beneath the blue

and freeway exit signs that point the way
toward God. Airplanes roar, saying nothing new.
Don't *waste this time*, I think, while palm trees sway.
I know we're lost, but can't think what to say.

Plonk

It was so nice to hear your voice again
last night, as if all had never gone wrong.
While you were holding forth on Rukeyser,
I sipped my glass of Côtes du Rhône, and smiled.
Your virtuosity astonished me
when I first heard you read your poetry.

It was so nice to hear your voice again
as if forgiveness weren't impossible.
While you were holding forth on Rukeyser,
I poured the Côtes du Rhône you gave me down
the drain. Your genius astonished me
when I first read your poetry in bed.

It was so nice to read your poetry
again, as if poetry could heal wounds.
While you were holding forth on Dickinson,
I thought of Rukeyser, and what you'd said
when we were drinking undistinguished wine
in Spain. Starched napkins spoke formality.

It was so nice to be in love with you
that way, as if poetry were a kind
of healing love. While you were holding forth,
I drank the table wine and laughed. I thought
you were like Rukeyser, or Dickinson—
brilliant, despite our drunken state, and fierce.

It was so nice to be with you, old friend.
Depression, migraines, breast cancer—and loss.
While you were holding forth on god-knows-what,
I knew I couldn't comfort you. Instead,
I wrote poetry that wasn't so good,
in forms that couldn't compensate for truth.

It was so nice to be with you in France,
before it all went so terribly wrong.
I was embarrassed when, too weak in French,
I asked in Spanish for the wine list. You
seemed vaguely annoyed, yet held forth on AIDS.
You ordered marrow bones and buttered toast.

It was so nice to be with you again,
if only briefly, and only on the page.
I still think of you when the waiter brings
the bottle of red wine, uncorks it, pours,
and looks at me for my approval. Yes,
I want to say, bring us another glass.

Views of Heaven

A storm passed through last night, leaving a mess
of sodden leaves and branches flung across

the yard. Amazing, how we two survived:
it's not just that before we realized

the truth, we could have been betrayed like him,
that college kid who played the violin

before he jumped, the George Washington Bridge
stretched out above him like the shining edge

of heaven; it's uncanny that no one
infected us when, half-drunk and alone,

we found ourselves in the East Village dark.
We'd crossed that same bridge; entering New York,

we felt so hopeful. Years since then, and still
I don't quite understand the reasons you'll

cook your pancakes without a recipe,
or keep the thermostat at sixty-three

all winter long, or say you love me when
you're tardy meeting me someplace, again.

I say I love you too, though I prefer
a simple omelet to pancakes, and turn

the thermostat back up to seventy.
Remarkable, that we don't starve, or freeze;

that spring will come again, and seem so late
like you, so joyous and never contrite.

We're in the middle age we might have never
had, old enough that we can start to savor

the seasons, memories, what seems our fate—
this love, that seems too plain to incite hate,

too commonplace to be worth killing for.
Yet I'd die to keep you safe. Never fear:

storms come, and bring their opportunity
to do another chore together, see

the world for what it really is. I look
at you, and think that even as you rake

these broken twigs and shattered leaves, I'm yours,
and you're the heaven I'm still rising toward.

Paternity

1.

I hear you outside laughing with their kids,
while farther off, a neighbor mows his lawn.
This morning, I watched you dream: your eyelids'
quick telegraphic flickering, while dawn

composed its own impossibilities.
I tried to enter that nice family
I know you want us to become. I see
you laughing with our son, who's reached your knees

in height. Impossibly, he looks like both
of us: his eyes are green like mine, his chin
is dimpled just like yours. You dream his birth,
you dream him running on a perfect lawn,

you dream me somewhere inside proud of him
while making sandwiches for lunch. I hear
you call to him, but when you say his name
you suddenly awaken, as if fear,

my fear, had clutched your heart. You're laughing now,
the neighbors' kids like those we'll never have.
I am more envious than I am proud:
you, perfect father; me, the missing half.

2.

Revision: outside, laughing, asking them
about their kids. Inside, I try to write.
This morning, watching you dream, I glimpsed him:
it was our son, emerging from the night,

half-formed in your half-smile, dancing in your
eyelids' fluttering. I tried hard to enter,
but in your dream I wasn't anymore.
Somewhere, a lawn mower began to sputter.

Yet there he was, our son, his eyes a green
I couldn't recognize, his dimpled chin
like yours. I knew it was your perfect dream.
I started dreaming too: yes, I loved him,

since he was my son too. You mowed the lawn,
while I made sandwiches I cut in half.
I served you lunch, but didn't know his name.
He looked at me as though I didn't have

a soul. When we awoke, I knew my sin.
You looked at me with such tremendous hurt
I thought I might not ever write again.
You, perfect father; me, my missing words.

The Massage

The neon strokes of Chinese characters
exclaimed the ancient city's endlessness.
Beijing at night: how much we cannot know,
how little we will ever understand.
For supper, jellyfish and giant clam,
profundities we couldn't contemplate;
and afterward, the acrobatic show
in which a tiny woman log-rolled you
(compliant "dear guest" from the audience)
teeteringly in an enormous urn,
her stocky legs splayed heavenward as if
she'd given birth to spectacle itself.
Arriving at the club, our hosts seemed pleased
our drunken acquiescence to their plans
allowed them to go on delighting us.
Your nakedness as we undressed seemed new,
redemptive and miraculous again,
the marble dressing room at once austere
and sexual, our hairy bodies crude
amid the sallow skin of Chinese men.
We put on skimpy bathrobes made of silk,
then padded down a mirrored corridor
past fake Venuses, and velvet-covered doors
whose mysteries we left inviolate.
Part-library, part-sanatorium,
the night's adventure would be ending here.
The girls were not beautiful. Clad in white,
they kept their firm caresses to our feet:
the scent of almond oil mixed with sweat,
their long black hair in loosely woven braids,
we wondered what price had been paid for them,
and whether we could be forgiven for
if only briefly thinking of forsaken

Mary Magdalene, suffering as much
for our same sins. If what we felt was shame
it was impossible to speak; if it
was grace, it remains imponderable.

On the Anniversary of the Terrorist Attacks

Someday, you may end up all alone.
As insidiously as September,
as pointlessly as writing poems,

as gradually as passing clouds are gone—
but when it happens, you'll remember.
Someday, you could end up all alone.

You will remember waiting for the phone
to ring, his voice familiar and tender,
and your wanting to write another poem

about the joy of him simply coming home,
dependability some kind of wonder.
Someday, you see, you will be all alone.

It should not be a shock, not entirely unknown.
He was never always your defender.
You have written many pointless poems.

What did you love best? How the light shone
in his eyes? Take-out Mexican not planned for?
Thinking that you'd never be alone?

Yet still, it stings, his black hair in the comb,
no tangled, warmed-up sheets to crawl under.
Instead, you'll have to write this pointless poem
someday, when you end up all alone.

Interrogative

That view out over the Golden Gate Bridge—
why couldn't it be

scythes clearing a meadow obscured by fog?
Why couldn't you be

here with me again, watching these hawks circle?
Why couldn't they be

some kind of portent? You said miracles
are what shouldn't be,

that I should stop hoping. Sage and wild fennel,
why can't you be

less sweet, why? Our footsteps echo through tunnels,
which couldn't be

a better metaphor: abandoned fort.
Why couldn't we

be more defenseless? "I left my heart,"
(it couldn't be!)

"in San Francisco," croons the radio.
Why couldn't we be

happy there? I'll tell you what we both know:
It wasn't meant to be.

Dreams

Some poets have dreams. Keats dreamed of beauty
regularly, while for Dickinson dreams
were a form of loneliness, or love.

Once I dreamed of becoming famous, like
Michael Chabon, whose novel, *Mysteries
of Pittsburgh*, was made into a movie.

The movie didn't do very well, but
it starred Peter Sarsgaard. I dream of him
regularly, out of loneliness, or

love. I dream I will meet him someday, that
he will star in the movie adapted
from my poetry. Somehow, we'll end up

in bed, and he will tell me all his dreams.
Auden was too urbane to dream, but damn
he was so good he never needed fame,

even if he did meet Queen Elizabeth.
What are dreams but palaces we don't own,
like beauty, or love? Sweetheart, come to bed.

The Golden Age of Venetian Painting

Champagne brunch, Tintoretto;
      afterward, you were terse.
Nymphs pursued through meadows,
      then raped by metaphors—
you loved me once with passion,
      not all that differently.
Your reasons, my emotions
      consumed what ached in me.

Gold coins fell in a shower;
      a swan trumpeted by;
I saw you in my mirror
      instead of me. So why
do we now act like children
      pretending not to know?
You ask too many questions.
      Your answer's always no.

The work grows dark, unfocused.
      As the great painter aged,
his colors grew more raucous.
      So does your uncorked rage
at this, my latest failure:
      not recognizing us,
your eyes, my sense of humor,
      our souls. We can't reverse

our half-wished dissolution.
      Too much is said, too much
not inadvertent pollution
      blights the other's warm touch.
We drive home from the city,
      those paintings well-placed wounds.
Your gaze is without pity;
      my longing, without bounds.

Shared

Like cigarettes stubbed out in ashtrays, trees
crowd round these blighted ponds: dead, gray, askew.
The whole world seems to be looking at you
as you pick your way carefully toward me.
It's always this way with remorse: it needs
to take away everything, even light,
even beauty, even the brief delight
that comes from owning our trivial deeds.
A chill wind rises, rattling the leaves
remaining on the brittle branches. Once,
years earlier, in the dumb radiance
of youth, we came here, if not to believe,
then to ask ourselves if we could become
what the other wanted so desperately.
You picked your way carefully toward me,
and I still remember the quiet hum
of countless insects flitting in the sun,
and the occasional calls of small birds
whose eloquence was more than any words.
We knew nothing about love between men,
but these ponds shimmered anyway, and life
seemed no less improbable or unsafe.
You kissed me tentatively. In your face,
I saw what has always been my belief:
that somehow we too entered paradise.
Years later, here we are again. The place
is dead, the trees poisoned by human waste,
the dumped chemicals of our avarice.
It was never really all about us;
I know that now as you look in my face
and see what I hope is some of God's grace.
The wind blows again: cold, anonymous,
yet not quite silent. You reach for my hand.

Together we return from memory,
I to your same smile, you to what in me
you seek. We don't believe; we understand.

Within

According to them, I contain too much,
those inner voices that will not shut up.
Internalized anxieties compete
for space with nobler inmates like the soul.
Imagination mingles waywardly
in there; distracted by a bird in flight,
I crashed into a tree while skiing once
and was reminded of my skeleton.
Of course, there are the poets' multitudes
who wish to sing at once, their memories
mistaken sometimes for my own, and then
these generations in my DNA,
discrediting the humors that were once
all we could glean of our trapped viscera.
It could be said that we are also made
of empty space, interstices of cells,
and deeper still, the yawning chasms where
electrons buzz beyond their proton pairs.
Such distances dissolve when we make love;
with you inside me we are both alone
and never so completely understood.
Yet still when we are tortured we will bleed,
the precious stuff of life released as if
what we call tears were truly ecstasy
itself, unquenchable, immeasurable,
and utterly impossible to hold within.

Love Song for Love Songs

A golden age of love songs and we still
can't get it right. Does your kiss really taste
like buttercream? To me, the moon's bright face
was neither like a pizza pie nor full;
the Beguine began, but my eyelid twitched.
"No more I love you's," someone else assured
us, pouring out her heart, in love (of course)—
what bothers me the most is that high-pitched,
undone whine of "Why am I so alone?"
Such rueful misery is closer to
the truth, but once you turn the lamp down low,
you must admit that he is still the one,
and baby, baby he makes you so dumb
you sing in the shower at the top of your lungs.

Poem Written at 5 AM on the Sweetness of Life

I woke to you encircled in my arms.
You faced away from me; in the half-light
it seemed you carried me toward what you dreamed.
I studied the back of your ear, but heard
nothing. I trusted that wherever you
were taking me was someplace free of fear.

What the Dead See

I wonder what the dead see back on earth.
The living play beach volleyball, dine on quiche.
The dead recall the quiet before birth.

The living play: Christmas near the roaring hearth,
feasting on joy, oblivious to ash.
I wonder what the dead see back on earth,

whether they are watching us, full of wrath,
or if instead it is regret, the wish
it weren't so quiet waiting for rebirth.

The living seem forgetful. We are both
voracious and yet limited by flesh.
We wonder if the dead look back at earth

as if our antics were all that were worth
revisiting. We harken to each crash,
afraid to think the quiet before birth

could someday yet engulf us. As will death.
And so the living play and feast and clash,
and wonder what the dead see back on earth.

If they are watching us watch fireworks,
what must concern them is our headlong rush,
how we are only quiet before birth,

how we forget. So merciless is truth
when we have disavowed grace. Hush, then, hush:
Let us ponder the quiet before birth,
let us wonder what the dead see back on earth.

Sestina in Red

There are six stories humans recognize.
Just six. The story in which boy meets girl.
The story someone once tried to invent.
The story critics see within the story.
The story of "Little Red Riding Hood."
The story nobody ever forgets.

There is another one, which I forget.
Look in my eyes, see what you recognize.
I'm the lost boy, Little Red Riding Hood—
I'm the little boy who thinks he's a girl.
The teacher doesn't understand my story.
"A story is not something to invent,"

a famous critic declared. We invent
excuses, we memorize lines, forget
them later. Always the same damn story:
Boy meets girl, boy loses girl—recognize
the pattern here?—boy realizes girl
was never his Little Red Riding Hood.

Big, bad wolves eat Little Red Riding Hood
in a version of the story I invent.
Or, the big bad wolf is really a girl!
The story everyone always forgets
is like the standard form we recognize.
Recall there is a story in the story;

or, every lie is an attempted story.
Our heroine Little Red Riding Hood
must pay for the lies we won't recognize.
The rape metaphor the critic invents
is like the memories we can't forget.
We tell the same story to little girls:

Once upon a time there was a bad girl
who tried to tell her side of the story.
"Please," she implored, "you must never forget."
I pretend I'm Little Red Riding Hood
so I can get lost in the woods, invent
the wolf so I don't have to recognize

truths we'd all like to forget. The wise girl
will recognize it's just that same old story
Little Red Riding Hood didn't invent.

The Destruction of the Temples of Machu Picchu

That such a place could possibly exist
terrifies the Spaniards who are the first
to weigh its splendor. In gold, they see lust;
in strange rites, evil born of jungle mist—

another god, more powerful than just.
That night, they pray together with the priest,
and ask why Christ would let this place exist.
The Spaniards speak terror. They're not the first

to be struck dumb by pride's undoubting fist.
By dawn, they know it must be done. In haste
they slaughter a thousand girls, then lay waste
to awe. They say none else were once so blessed;
they swear such a place never did exist.